Top 30 Delicious Smoothies That Burns Fat, Increases Your Metabolism and Keeps You In Shape

Learn to be a Smoothie master with 25+ veteran recipes and exclusive peek into the nutritional values to help you Sip up and Slim Down!

Introduction

Popularly known as a Smoothy, and Smoothie, these are the trendiest beverages of our era as well our ancestors'. From mocktails to cocktails, smoothies can be part of any lifestyle. In fact, prolonged and religious use of smoothies will help your body shed weight and gain healthy cells rhythmically. In fact, being fibrous and wholesome, smoothies are the ideal option if you want to have an effortless, efficient diet plan wherein the health quotient of your body, increases.

The book will help you understand why smoothies are the ultimate solution to weight loss diets and how to be a Smoothie expert with an enviable figure! With my handpicked smoothie recipes and nutritional overview, you will know everything you need to start your natural and 100% effective diet.

If you're ready to learn, our in-depth analysis and exclusive smoothies that will help you hack the secret of your weight loss too!

Good Luck and Get ready to Sip in and Slim out!

Contents

Chapter 7 5 Hacks of the Best Dinner Smoothies

Conclusion

YOUR FREE GIFT

As a way of showing my gratitude towards your purchase, I'm offering my Epic-5-Day Smoothy Weight Loss Diet

I assure you that this is the same diet plan that I had scribbled on my first fitness book and the same that freed hundreds of my clients from the burdening fat issue. It is a very simple diet plan, based on the same recipes that this book contains but in a very structured manner for the 5 days and works wonders

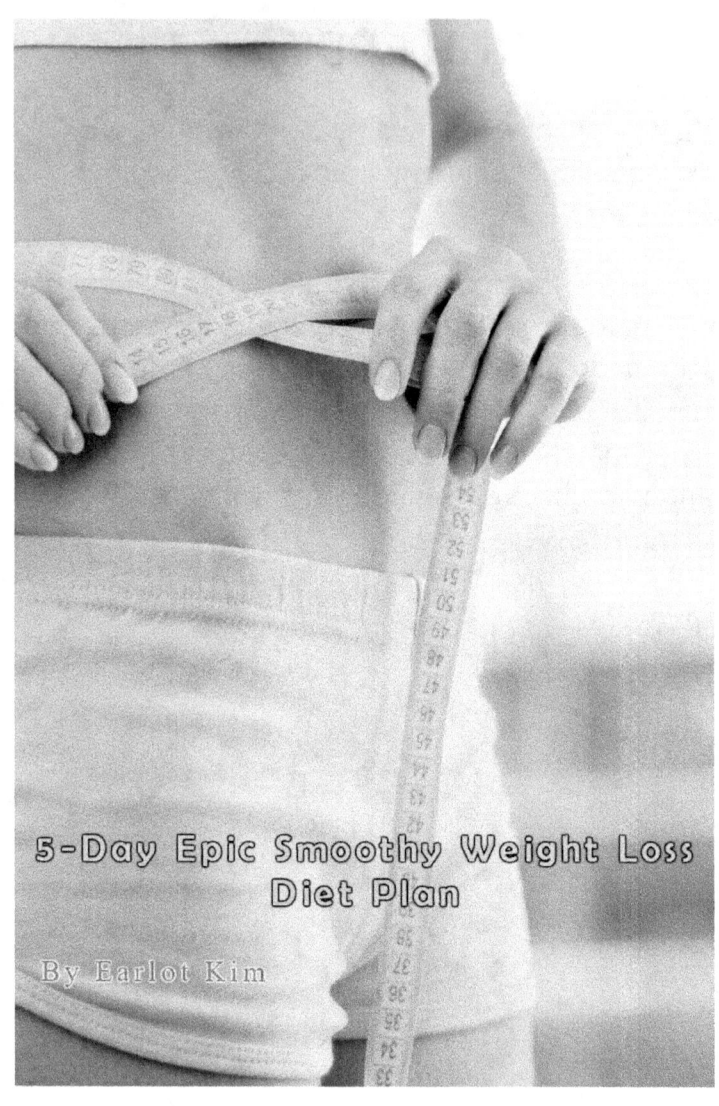

5-Day Epic Smoothy Weight Loss Diet Plan

By Earlot Kim

http://smoothydietplan.gr8.com/

Chapter 1
Everything You Need To Know About Weight Loss Smoothies

Do you know the difference between a juice and a smoothie? The thin line separating the two is made up of fibres. Seriously, it is! The former pumps the juice out of a fruit after removing the fibres, while the latter simply bends a whole fruit. When you eat the juice of a whole fruit, the amount of energy necessary to break down the pulp is negligible, as the juicer has done the job already.

So what is a smoothie?

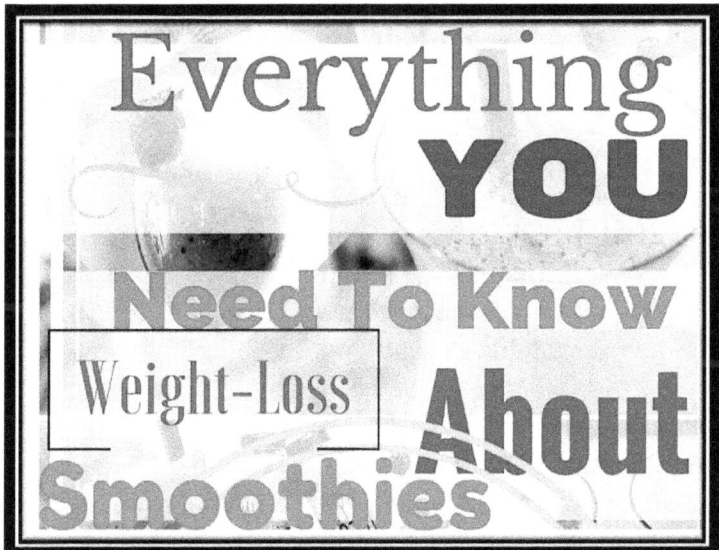

What are Weight Loss Smoothies Made of?

Smoothies are an ideal substitute for meals and not just another beverage. An ideally healthy smoothie that is beneficial to your stomach must have the following five core things:

- **Liquid**: Water, Milk, Coconut Water, Green Tea or Juice
- **Choice of Fruit or Vegetable:**
    - Pick one creamy fruit: Mango, Avocado, Banana, Peach or Pear
    - Pick one Non-creamy fruit: Pineapple, orange, berries, melon, dry fruits or apples
    - Pick one Vegetable: Spinach, Kale, Lettuce, Bitter gourd, Cucumber, Carrot, Kale, Squash and sweet potato.
- **To Dilute or To Thicken:** Ice, Yoghurt, Curd, Nuts, Tofu and Yoghurt (Low-fat or Greek)
- **For Flavour**: Honey, Vanilla, Agave, Cinnamon, Nutmeg, Cocoa and Dates are ideal for additional flavors.
- **Protein and Taste**: Apart from flavours if you're looking for a healthy power play in your weight loss smoothie, try wheat gram, flax, soy, spirulina and hemp proteins in your smoothie.

Why use these ingredients?

Our nature is filled with many elixirs such that fruit and vegetables are abundant in minerals and vitamins. In fact, for different geographies, the nutrition quotient of the fruits and vegetables might vary. Here is a guide to help you understand the ideal universal ratio for a smoothie:

- **_Liquid:_** _1 Part_
- **_Fruit/ Vegetable:_** _2 Parts_
- **_Thickener/ Creaminess_**_: 1 Parts_
- **_Flavour:_** _As needed_
- **_Nutrition Add-ins:_** _1 Part_

Nevertheless, all fruits and ingredients always differ in their nutritional facts depending on its topography.

Things You Need To Start Making Weight Loss Smoothies

Before beginning the Smoothie diet, you must have an idea about the ideal picks for a weight loss smoothie as well as mixing it to suit your personal tastes. The golden rule before beginning on Smoothie Prep is:

Always add liquid to your blender first!

Here's the list of fruits, vegetables, sweeteners, thickeners, flavours and nutritional substances that you need in a weight loss smoothie.

- **Chia Seeds**: Mainly for the nutritional value, Chia seeds fill the appetite apart from being a rich source of protein. They also expand once in the stomach and works as an appetite suppressor.
- **Banana:** Creamy with sugary flavour can give you the necessary boost for metabolism due to the presence of potassium and Vitamin B.
- **Strawberry:** For flavour, core taste and fibre, strawberries are ideal for weight loss as they help in increasing the metabolism.
- **Coconut Milk**: Adds creaminess and flavour to the smoothie if you want to displace milk in your smoothie.

- **Yoghurt**: Burns fat, adds creaminess and flavour to the smoothie.
- **Cocoa:** Appetite suppressant and protein source for feeling full for longer hours
- **Almond Milk:** Protein source to decrease appetite and increase the feeling of being full
- **Honey**: Flavour, Sweetener and minerals that boost weight loss through healthy digestion and metabolism
- **Flaxseed**: Fibrous and highly absorbent to fluids, adding these in the smoothie will help in digestion and energy equivalent to a meal
- **Spinach**: A rich nutrient source, spinach is highly antioxidant to help fight the free radical damages of your body and skin to provide for the health and smooth digestion.
- **Cabbage**: Vitamin C source, which is fibrous and adds flavour to the smoothie
- **Cinnamon:** Flavour as well as digestion aid that increases the feeling of fullness and boosts energy in the body
- **Mango:** Suppresses appetite and is popular as a meal maker.
- **Blackberries:** Flavour, Sweetener and a healthy antioxidant to keep your body and less hungry through the day
- **Raspberries:** Antioxidants and a boost of Energy
- **Blueberries:** Rich in Vitamins and antioxidants
- **Green Apples:** Fibrous and Rich in Vitamins, Green apples keep the bodily metabolisms active and healthy
- **Kiwi:** Ideal for weight-loss, these are loaded with nutrients, fibre and tropical fresh flavour.

- **Avocado:** Decreases appetite and is a rich source of fibres.
- **Flaxseed Oil:** PUFAs (polyunsaturated fatty acids) like Omega 3 is present in Flaxseed oil to cut down the binge eating and remain full for longer time.
- **Peach:** Used as a Sweetener and for flavour
- **Orange:** Vitamins and detoxification of the body
- **Lemon:** Hub of minerals, Vitamins and Protein such that it detoxifies your body with 0% cholesterol
- **Hemp Protein:** High in iron, calcium and null cholesterol, hemp proteins are ideal for weight loss smoothies that displace meals.
- **Spirulina**: This is equivalent to a whole meal and is made from cyanobacterium and has extremely high counts of potassium and Sodium with least cholesterol

Chapter 2
5 Easy Smoothies To Sip Up & Slim Down

Being a versatile beverage, you can add the exotic nuttiness or oriental greenery to your smoothies suiting your hallmark tastes whenever you want that exotic zest on your palette. Here's my exclusive list of smoothies that are picked out for their low-calorie quotients and high stamina assurance. I have personally made and consumed it over the years that I am not the lone advocate of these recipes, but my kids and friends too.

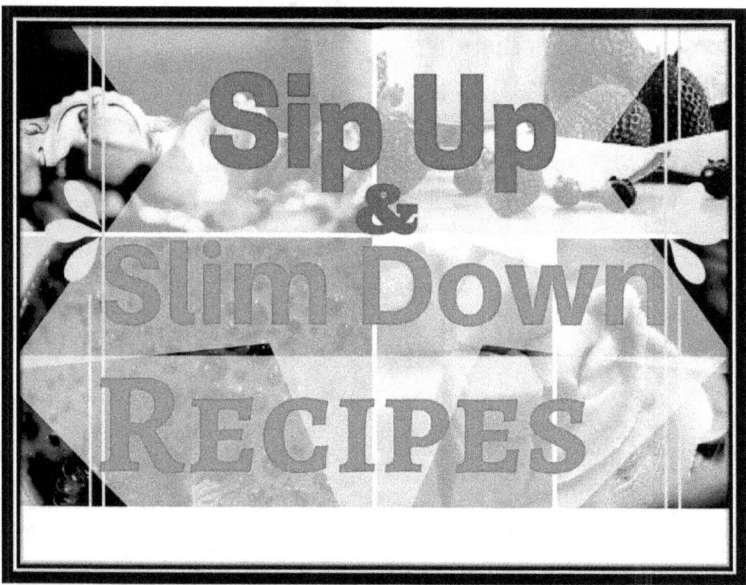

Get ready to Sip Up and Slim Down!

- ***Mango 'n' Avocado With a dash of Lime***
  Refreshing, energizing and detoxifying for mornings and weary evenings

Ingredients You Will Need

Avocado: One
Mango: One
Lime: One or Two
Low Fat Yoghurt: 8 Ounces
Mint: 1 Tablespoon
Ice/ Milk: As needed
Honey: As needed but not more than one spoonful

How Do you Prepare it?

Mix honey and lime and pour into the blender. Add the core ingredients. Smoothen it up!

Nutritional Fact

This Smoothie is ideal for weight loss s it adds up to nothing but under 300 Calories while boosting your energy and suppressing hunger.

- ### <u>Blueberries in Soy Milk 'n' Honey</u>

  Also known as the Canadian smoothie, blueberries smoothies are ideally baby pink in colour and nutritiously akin to the best natural health drink.

Ingredients You Will Need

Blueberries: 1 Cup
Soy Milk: 1 Cup
Honey: As needed
Ice: As needed
Banana: For Creaminess

How do you Prepare it?

Add liquids into the blender. Add sliced core ingredients. Blend it all. Add ice cubes. Blend again until smooth and creamy.

Nutritional Fact
*Perfect for weight loss, the smoothie is loaded with
Potassium, fibres and 'Zero' on Cholesterol with
under 500 Calories.*

- **Peanut Butter Berry with Yoghurt and
  Honey in Banana**
  Popularly known as Peanut Butter berry, when
  mixed with different flavours, the smoothie
  produces unique and diverse tastes.

Ingredients You Will Need
Blueberries: 1 Cup
Yoghurt: 2 Cups
Peanut Butter: 3 Spoonful+
Ice: As needed
Banana: 1 Cup
Honey: As needed

How do you Prepare it?
Add the liquids first and blend well. Add the core
ingredients and blend again. Now, add the ice and
blend until smooth.

Nutritional Fact
*With less than 300 calories, a peanut butter
smoothie has fewer than 5mg Cholesterol and high
proteins as well as least sugars.*

- **Coconut Water in Strawberries 'n 'Chia
  seeds**
  Served chilled, this is an ideal tropical beverage for
  a weary evening of hunger and fatigue.

Ingredients You Will Need

Coconut Water: 1.5 Cups
Strawberries: 2 Cups
Chia Seeds: As needed
Banana: As needed for Creaminess
Ice: As needed
Honey: Up to two spoonful

How do you Prepare it?

In an order of coconut water first, add strawberries, bananas and the remnant ingredients except for chia seeds. Blended it all and pour it into your glass. Top with chia seeds and consume after refrigeration.

Nutritional Fact

With just 33 Calories in 1 Cup of coconut water, the total calories of the smoothie is brought down to under 150 and is ideally packed with potassium and null Cholesterol.

- **<u>Yummy Almond Milk in Kiwi and Spirulina</u>**
  A green smoothie, this is filled with a diet filled with proteins, energy and powers such that one glass full of Yummy Almond Milk will fill your dinner or breakfast well!

Ingredients You Will Need

Almond Milk: Half Cup
Spirulina: One Spoonful
Kiwi: Two Whole Kiwis
Honey: As needed
Ice: As needed

How do you Prepare it?

Add everything in a blender beginning with the liquid and blend until you achieve the desired consistency. Add the ice and blend again.

Nutritional Fact

Weighing less than 50 Calories, this smoothie is the epitome the pink of health with dietary fibres alongside null cholesterol.

Chapter 3
Five Revitalizing Breakfast Smoothies

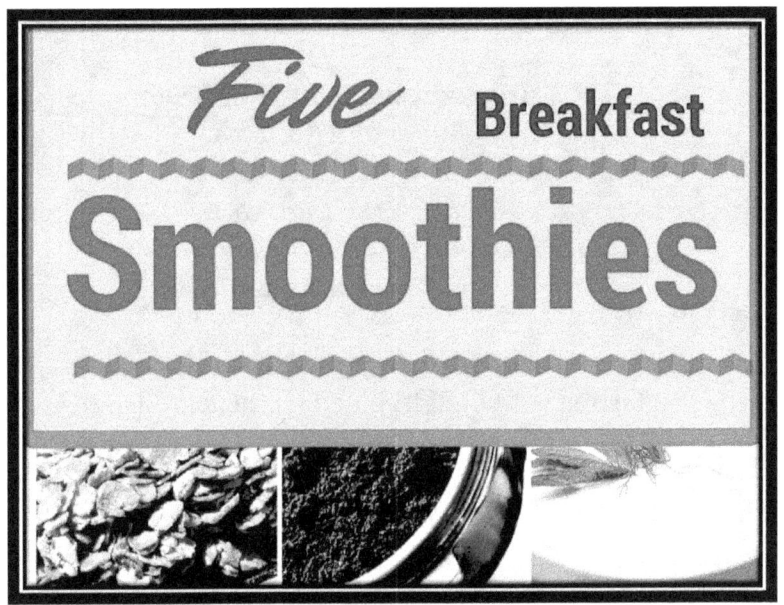

- **Dewy Sunrise Coffee**

Ingredients You Will Need
Coffee: As needed
Milk: Half Cup
Honey: As needed
Cinnamon: As needed
Ice: As needed
Beginning with milk, blend all your ingredients in a blender until it is smooth. Now add the ice and blend again until desired.

With 66 Calories, this is a power packed smoothie with an average count of >10 mg cholesterol and high proteins.

- ## Banana in Rejuvenating Ginger

Ingredients You Will Need
Banana: 2 (wedged)
Honey: As needed
Ginger: Half Cup (Grated)
Flaxseeds: 2 Spoonful
Ice/ Water: As needed

How do you prepare?
Starting with liquids, blend all the ingredients until smooth.

Ideal for burning stomach fat, this smoothie has less than 250 calories and is loaded with proteins to keep you feeling full for 2-3 hours.

- ## Oats with Blueberries

Ingredients You Will Need
Oats: Half Cup (prepared)
Honey: As needed
Blueberries: 1 Cup
Mint: As needed

How do you prepare?
Blend all of the above until smooth. Add ice for chilled effect.
Gluten free ideal breakfast smoothie, this purple smoothie has a total calorie value of 179-230 Calories.

- **<u>Cranberry Sauce in Yoghurt</u>**

Ingredients You Will Need
Leftover Cranberry Sauce (frozen): 8 (Cubes)
Yoghurt: Quarter Cup
Honey: As needed

How do you prepare?
Put all the ingredients in a blender and blend until the desired texture is achieved.

A delicious breakfast for camping as well as office, the smoothie has a total calorie value of 150-200.

- **<u>Green Tea in Agave and Yoghurt</u>**

Ingredients You Will Need
Green Tea: Half Cup
Ice: As needed (More for Iced Green Tea Smoothie)
Agave: One Spoon
Banana: One Wedged
Yoghurt: Half Cup
Honey: As needed

How do you prepare?
Mix all the ingredients except ice in a blender. Add ice one everything else is blended and serve chilled.

Having less than 300 Calories, the above smoothie is ideal for breakfast part of weight-loss than a milk shake.

Chapter 5
Favourite Five Lunch Smoothies

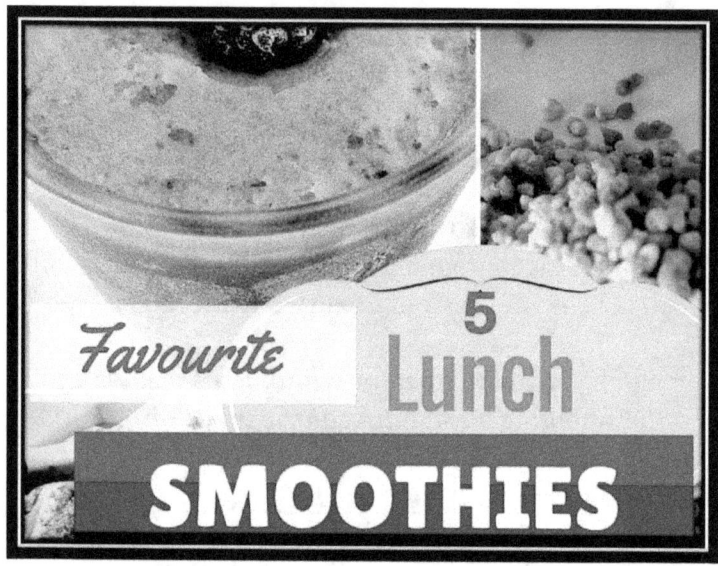

- **<u>Green For Health Mint, Spinach and Parsley Smoothie</u>**

Ingredients You Will Need
Mint: 1 Spoonful
Parsley: Quarter Cp
Spinach: Half Cup
Honey: As needed
Yoghurt: For Creaminess, as needed

How do you prepare?
Blend all the ingredients together. Prepare in batches and keep to have once every two hours.

With > 200 Calories, this smoothie is ideal to satisfy for a diet lunch.

- ### Honey Bee Pollen with oats and Dates

  ### Ingredients You Will Need
  Bee Pollens: 1 Spoonful
  Oats: Half Cup
  Ice: As needed
  Dates: As needed (Not more than 3 for 1 Cup of Smoothie)

  ### How do you prepare?
  Blend all the ingredients in a blender, except bee pollen and ice. Pause and add ice to blend again. Add bee pollen and refrigerate again.

  The smoothie has a total calorie count of 230 and is rich in Vitamin A, C and K apart from proteins.

- ### Double Decker Berry Delight in Pineapple Juice

  ### Ingredients You Will Need
  Pineapple juice: 1 Cup
  Honey: As needed
  Kiwis: 2 Cups
  Strawberries: 1 Cup
  Avocado: 1 Cup

  ### How do you prepare?
  Blend Kiwis, Pineapple juice, avocado and honey together. Pour it into your smoothie glasses, to fill it half. Blend Strawberries and honey in the blender now. Pour this over earlier blend. Garnish with chia seeds or bee pollen and enjoy your hearty meal!

Being under 350 calories, this complete meal will satisfy you and engage in efficient metabolic activities to suppress your hunger for the next 2-3 hours.

- **Tropical Raspberry Coconut Gratings**

  ### Ingredients You Will Need
  Raspberries: 1 Cup
  Frozen Banana: 1 Cup (Cubed)
  Honey: As needed
  Coconut Gratings: Half Cup
  Ice: As need

  ### How do you prepare?
  Blend in all the ingredients except ice, which is added, ideally at last.

  With a good calories count of 454, this smoothie is the ultimate elixir for the weary worker needing a wholesome lunch smoothie.

- **Spinach, Kale and Pineapple for Gluten Free Lunch**

  ### Ingredients You Will Need
  Spinach: Half Cup
  Banana Chunks: Half Cup
  Kale: Quarter Cup
  Almond Butter: 1 Tablespoons
  Ice: As needed
  Honey: As needed

  ### How do you prepare?

Take all the ingredients except ice and blend it. Pause, now add ice and blend until a smooth consistency is achieved.

Under 250 Calories, this smoothie is also a stamina booster for diet lunches, as it is high in sodium and proteins.

Chapter 6
Super Easy Ten Snacks and Dessert Smoothies

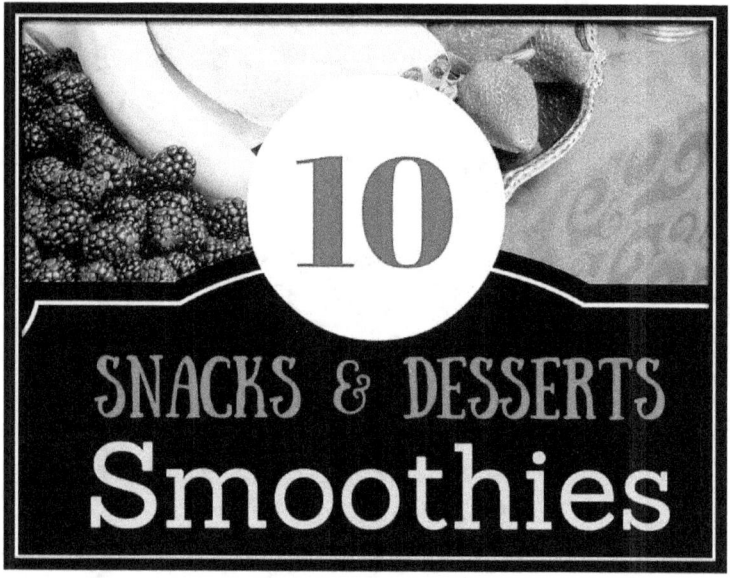

- ## <u>After Workout</u>

Ingredients You Will Need
Kale: 1.5 Cups
Frozen Pineapple Cubes: 1 Cup
Spirulina: Half teaspoon
Chia Seeds: As needed
Honey: As needed
Yoghurt: Half Cup
Ice: As needed

How do you prepare?
Mix the yoghurt, kale, pineapple cubes, spirulina and honey in a blender. Pause and add ice to blend

again. Now, add chia seeds and refrigerate to chill your exhaustion-off, post workout.

Calculated at 250-300 Calories, this recipe is appropriate for weight loss as it provides abundant proteins to keep the stamina up and hunger down!

- ### Ironing Up Indian Jal Jeera (Cumin in Water)

Ingredients You Will Need
Jaljeera/ Jaljira Powder (Cumin, Pepper, Mint, Black Salt): 2 Teaspoon
Ice: 2 Cups
Soda or Water: 1 Cup

How do you prepare?
Blend all the ingredients together and consume in one sip for a healthy and nourishing summer elixir!

The popular summer drink in India has the least Calories and is an ancient secret weight loss drink that quenches thirst and hunger while keeping the body charged!

- ### Spicy Butternut in Bananas as a Snack

Ingredients You Will Need
Ice: As needed
Butternut squash: 1 Cup (Steamed)
Frozen Soy Milk: Half Cup
Banana: One (Diced)
Honey: As needed

How do you prepare?
Blend all of the above until smooth and have it chilled

With less than 200 calories, this smoothie is a powerhouse of sodium and proteins.

- ## Green Apples Pie

Ingredients You Will Need
Green Apples:1 (diced)
Honey: As needed
Yoghurt: Half Cup
Banana: One (Diced)
Ice: As needed

How do you prepare?
Take all the ingredients except ice and smoothen it in a blender until the desired consistency is achieved.

With an overall calorie count lesser than 400, this smoothie has above 17.8g Protein to keep you full and alert.

- ## Pumpkin Tea Pie

Ingredients You Will Need
Almond Milk: Half Cup
Dry Tea leaves:1 Spoonful
Pumpkin pie: 2 spoonful
Frozen Banana: 1 Cup (Diced)

How do you prepare?

Put all the ingredients in a blender except dry tealeaves and blending until smooth. Add tea leaves to the smoothie and refrigerate it.

Being >300 calories, the smoothie has 8g+ fibres and is ideally packed with null cholesterol.

Desserts

- ## Healthy Cake Batter Glassed

Ingredients You Will Need
Ice: As needed
Yoghurt: Half Cup
Cake Mix: Half Cup
Spirulina: A Pinch
Honey: As needed

How do you prepare?
Add all the ingredients except ice in the blender to mix well. Add the ice at last and blend again to serve chilled.

Less than 250 calories and null cholesterol, this smoothie is loaded with proteins as well.

- ## Brownie in a Glass for dessert

Ingredients You Will Need
Almond Milk: 1 Cup
Frozen Banana: One (Diced)
Dates/ Honey: As needed

How do you prepare?

Blend all of the above until smooth and have it after refrigeration.

Ranging up to 180 calories, this is an ideal dessert for anyone craving sweets while on a weight-loss diet!

- **<u>Banana Bread in Walnuts</u>**

Ingredients You Will Need
Walnuts: 1 Cup
Water: 2 Cups
Frozen Banana: 1.5 Cups (Diced)
Honey: As needed
Nutmeg and Cinnamon: As needed

How do you prepare?
Make Walnut milk by soaking raw walnuts for 4+ hours and extracting nothing but the pulp. Blend all the ingredients sans ice in a blender. Pause and blend with ice until the desired consistency is noted.

Totalling > 300 Calories, this is staple smoothie with high protein (10g+) and fibres (6g+)

- **<u>Kiwi on Banana and Mint</u>**

Ingredients You Will Need
Kiwi: 2-3 (diced)
Frozen Banana: One cup (Diced)
Mint: One Teaspoon
Honey: As needed
Ice: As needed

How do you prepare?

Blend all ingredients except ice. Pause and blend with ice. Pour and Sip up!

Totalling up to 300 Calories, this smoothie is high on fibre (12g+) null on cholesterol.

- ### **Double Decker Super Strength Smoothie**

Ingredients You Will Need
Banana: One Cup (cubes)
Spirulina: 1 spoonful
Spinach: One Cup
Strawberries: One Cup (Diced)
Almond Milk: Half Cup
Honey: As needed
Ice: As needed

How do you prepare?
Add quarter cup of almond milk and blend bananas, spinach and honey with spirulina in the blender. Pour this into 3/4th of your smoothie cup. Now blend strawberries, quarter cup of almond milk, honey and ice. Pour this over the smoothie cup to fill it. Serve chilled!

The double-decker Super Strength Smoothie is less than 230 calories, with 1000+ grams of Potassium and sodium prevalent with high protein quotient.

Chapter 7
Five Hacks Of Dinner Smoothies

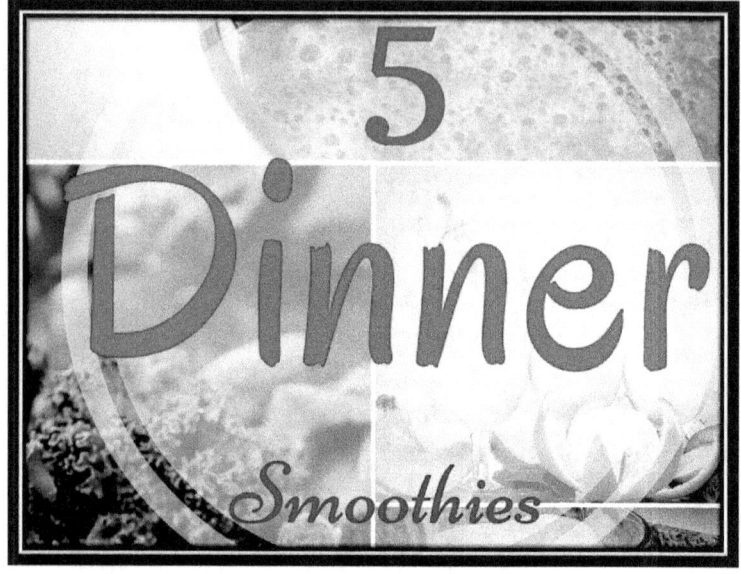

- ## Hemp in Spinach Smoothie

Ingredients You Will Need
Hemp Seeds: 1 Teaspoon (Powdered)
Spinach: Half Cup
Soy Milk: 1 Cup
Honey: As needed

How do you prepare?
Blend all of the above until you achieve a smooth consistency.

A dash of lime to the above will also help in detoxifying your body. The smoothie has less than 350 calories and is an ideal smoothie for weight loss dinners.

- ### Detox With Ginger, Pear and Kale

  #### Ingredients You Will Need
  Ginger Paste: Quarter Cup
  Lemon: 3 Teaspoon
  Pear Extracts: Half Cup
  Kale: Quarter Cup
  Honey: As needed
  Ice: As needed

  #### How do you prepare?
  Blend all the ingredients, in the order of liquids first to blend first. Pause, add the ice, and blend until the desired consistency is achieved.

  Rated less than 180 Calories this smoothie is an ideal dinner smoothie due to the incredible detoxification it provides to the body.

- ### Indian Lassi

  #### Ingredients You Will Need
  Yoghurt: 3 Cups
  Honey: As needed
  Ice: Half Cup

  #### How do you prepare?
  Blend yoghurt and honey until the smoothie has a no-grain consistency. Pause, add ice and continue blending until a smooth texture is achieved.

  Even though a filling meal, Indian Lassi has a calorie count of less than 160 units.

- ## **Green Smoothie**

Ingredients You Will Need
Lettuce: Half Cup
Frozen Cucumber: Half Cup
Kale: Quarter Cup
Cabbage: Quarter Cup
Honey: As needed

How do you prepare?
Add all of the above to a blender and blend until the desired consistency is achieved.

Most popular smoothie for weight-loss diet, having green vegetables and fruits with apt flavours cuts down your fat. This recipe has a calorie count of less than 100.

- ## **Vitamins Smoothie**

Ingredients You Will Need
Orange: Quarter Cup
Pineapple: Quarter Cup
Pappaya: Quarter Cup
Banana: Half (Diced)
Cinnamon: A pinch
Honey: As needed

How do you prepare?
Blend all of the above in a blender and serve chilled.

Having less than 250 calories and loaded with a power meal that will energize and repair your body, vitamins smoothie is the ideal dinner for weight loss diets.

YOUR FREE GIFT

As a way of showing my gratitude towards your purchase, I'm offering my Epic-5-Day Smoothy Weight Loss Diet

I assure you that this is the same diet plan that I had scribbled on my first fitness book and the same that freed hundreds of my clients from the burdening fat issue. It is a very simple diet plan, based on the same recipes that this book contains but in a very structured manner for the 5 days and works wonders

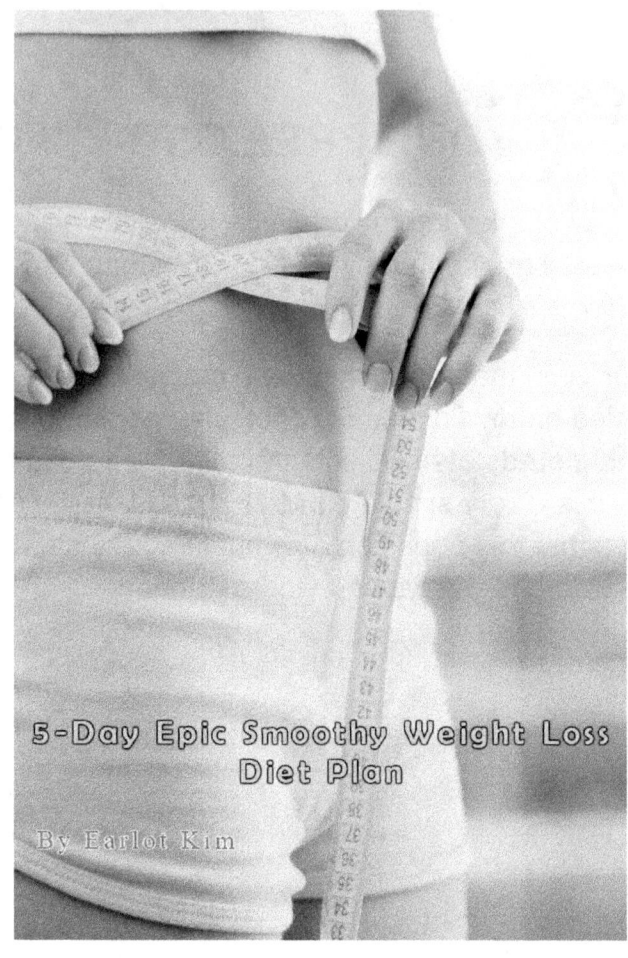

5-Day Epic Smoothy Weight Loss Diet Plan

By Earlot Kim

Conclusion

Thank you for downloading this book. Let nature bless you with its sweetest elixirs now that you know every untold secret to make a smoothie ...

I hope my expertise has helped you understand all sides of how elixir smoothies work on our bodies. There are smoothies that burden your body with more weight, while healthy smoothies like all of the above are strictly for weight loss.

When appropriately used, smoothies are elixirs. Now, that you have completed the book successfully, it is time to put your theories into practise. Pack up you kindle and head to the kitchen and begin your culinary capade with an exotic weight-loss recipe RIGHT NOW! Treat your family to a Smoothie Day once per week and feel the magic yourself!

Good Luck!

Finally, if you enjoyed this book, then I'd like to ask you for a favor, would you be kind enough to leave a review for this book on Amazon? It'd be greatly appreciated!

I love getting feedback from my readers and reviews on amazon really do make a difference. I read all my reviews and would really appreciate your thoughts.

Thank you
-Earlot